# Easy & ]
# Gluten-F

*Tasty & Creamy, Sweet & Savory Gluten-Free Snack Recipes That Taste Better Than "Normal Food"*

By Kira Novac

ISBN: 9781098596422

Copyright ©Kira Novac 2019

www.amazon.com/author/kira-novac

All rights reserved. No part of this publication may be reproduced, stored in a retrieval system, or transmitted, in any form or by any means, electronic, mechanical, photocopying, recording or otherwise, without the prior written permission of the author and the publishers.

The scanning, uploading, and distribution of this book via the Internet, or via any other means, without the permission of the author is illegal and punishable by law. Please purchase only authorized electronic editions, and do not participate in or encourage electronic piracy of copyrighted materials.

All information in this book has been carefully researched and checked for factual accuracy. However, the author and publishers make no warranty, expressed or implied, that the information contained herein is appropriate for every individual, situation or purpose, and assume no responsibility for errors or omission. The reader assumes the risk and full responsibility for all actions, and the author will not be held liable for any loss or damage, whether consequential, incidental, and special or otherwise, that may result from the information presented in this publication.

A physician has not written the information in this book. Before making any serious dietary changes, I advise you to consult with your physician first.

# Free Complimentary Recipe eBook

Thank you so much for taking an interest in my work!

As a thank you, I would love to offer you a free complimentary recipe eBook to help you achieve vibrant health. It will teach you how to prepare amazingly tasty and healthy gluten-free treats so that you never feel deprived or bored again!

As a special bonus, you will be able to receive all my future books (kindle format) for free or only $0.99.

**Download your free recipe eBook here:**

[http://bit.ly/gluten-free-desserts-book](http://bit.ly/gluten-free-desserts-book)

# GLUTEN-FREE, GUILT-FREE AND STRESS-FREE!

*Irresistible Gluten-Free Desserts, Snacks and Treats for Vibrant Health, Weight Loss and Longevity*

**KIRA NOVAC**

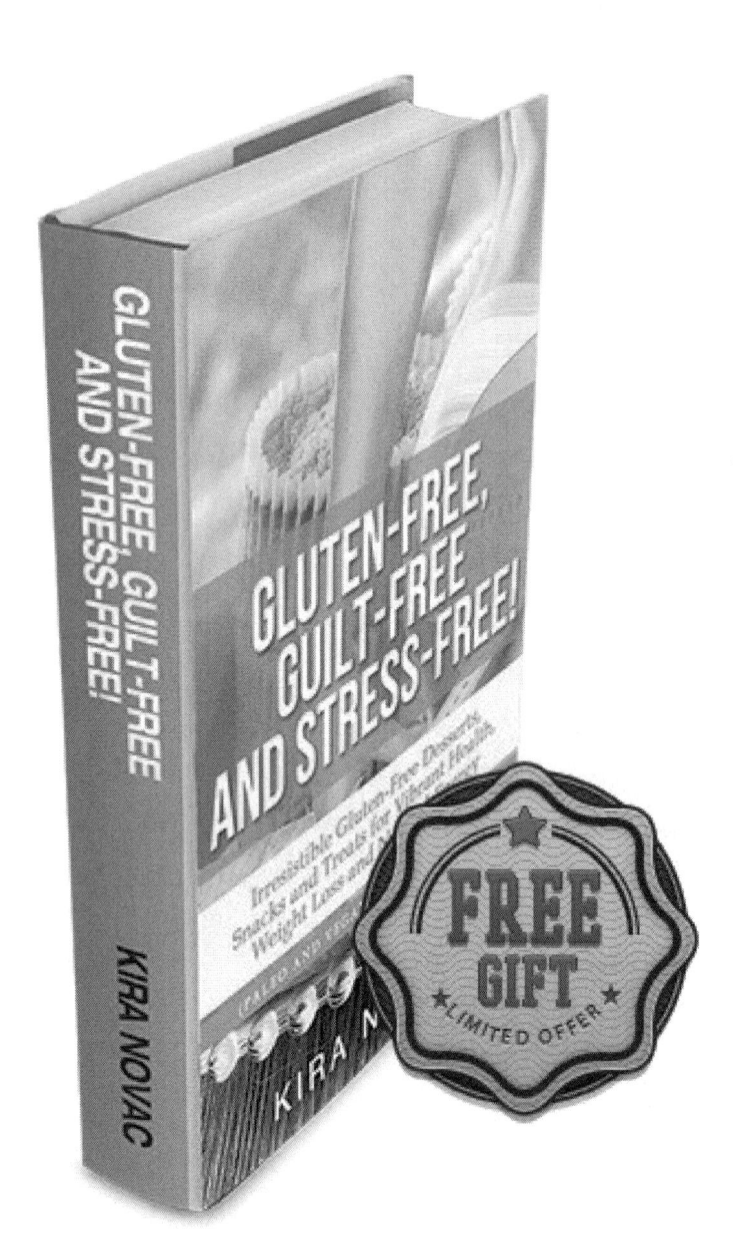

**FREE GIFT — LIMITED OFFER**

# Table of contents

Introduction .................................................................................. 1

    A Life of Gluten-Free Snacking ........................................... 1

    Where is Gluten Found? ....................................................... 3

    What Does Gluten DO? ......................................................... 3

    What Can I Eat? .................................................................... 5

    Extra Tips for Gluten Free Cooking ..................................... 7

    Celebrate the foods you can eat... ....................................... 8

The Recipes .................................................................................. 9

    Sweet Snacks ........................................................................ 9

        Jam Popovers .................................................................. 10

        Chunky Monkeys ........................................................... 12

        Fruit Bakes ..................................................................... 14

        Chocolate Bean Cake ..................................................... 16

        Citrus, Sultana and Polenta Slice ................................. 18

        Chestnut and Apricot Jam Muffins .............................. 20

        Gluten-Free Biscotti ...................................................... 22

        Chestnut Flour and Brown Sugar Shortbread Wedges ........... 25

        Peanut Oaties ................................................................. 27

        Ginger Cookies .............................................................. 29

        No Cook Rice Cake Bonanza! ....................................... 31

Gluten-Free Funnel Cakes.................................................................37

Brownies Gone Blonde......................................................................40

Popped Corn!.....................................................................................42

Ginger and Dark Chocolate Flapjack Cookies ........................45

Gluten Free Snack Bread..................................................................47

French Toasties (using the gluten-free snack loaf) ................49

Fruit Topped Bread (using the gluten-free snack loaf) ..........52

Baked Banana and Chocolate Fingers (using the gluten-free snack loaf)................................................................................................54

Fruity Kebabs ......................................................................................56

Fruit Scones.........................................................................................58

For the Fruit Spread..........................................................................60

Mug Cake Snacks...............................................................................62

Oat Apple Balls ..................................................................................65

Savoury Snacks......................................................................................67

Flaxseed Wraps ..................................................................................68

Chinese Prawn Snack Rolls............................................................71

Muffin Mugs .......................................................................................74

Courgette and Feta Cakes...............................................................78

Socca with an Herb Crust ..............................................................80

Baked Garlic Mushroom Bites .....................................................83

Sesame Seed Crackers .................................................................... 85

Parsnip and Rosemary Fries ........................................................... 87

Mini Pizza Bites ............................................................................... 89

Mozzarella Sticks ............................................................................ 92

Ricotta and Spinach Flatbread ....................................................... 94

Green Crisps ................................................................................... 97

Carrot Cornbread ............................................................................ 99

Savoury Pan Scones ..................................................................... 101

Bacon Salad Cups ......................................................................... 103

Cauliflower Wraps ......................................................................... 105

Cloud Bread Bakes ........................................................................ 107

Parmesan Funnel Cakes ............................................................... 109

Coconut Spiced Funnel Cakes ...................................................... 111

Greek Salad Kebab (using the gluten-free snack loaf) ............... 114

Toasted Welsh Rarebit (using the gluten-free snack loaf) ........ 116

Chicken Bombs and Chilli Dip ...................................................... 118

No-Cook Cracker Toppings Bonanza! .......................................... 120

Smokey Cauliflower Steak ........................................................... 124

Garlic Twists ................................................................................. 126

Smorgasbord ................................................................................. 129

Bacon and Broccoli Fritter ........................................................... 131

Energy Snacks ................................................................ 133

    3 Flavours of Energy ............................................... 134

    Coconut Bounce Balls ............................................. 136

    Middle Eastern Boost .............................................. 138

    Freezer Fuel ............................................................. 140

    Sticky Date Energy Bars ......................................... 142

    Tropical Energy Bars .............................................. 144

    Bike Bites ................................................................. 146

    Peanut Butter Energy Cups ................................... 148

    Apple Pie Energy Bars ............................................ 150

    Ginger Rush Bars .................................................... 152

    Fudge Brownie Energy Bar ................................... 154

    Nut Free Energy Balls ............................................ 156

Conclusion .................................................................... 159

To post an honest review ............................................ 161

Recommended Reading ............................................. 163

# Introduction

## *A Life of Gluten-Free Snacking*

Nowadays, many people are opting to choose a life of gluten-free living and this is not just because they have to. Various studies and theories are emerging that gluten may be responsible for a number of symptoms and medical conditions and there are many us who have found relief from certain health complaints when avoiding gluten in their diets.

1 in 100 people are a Coeliac. This means they have an auto-immune condition, where gluten can do irreparable damage to the body and cause bad health it they consume it. This is a medically confirmed condition and is usually diagnosed with a blood test and it is important to be followed up by a medical provider to ensure you are remaining fit and well.

Other people find they have an intolerance or sensitivity to gluten, where it causes bloating, weight gain, diarrhoea, tiredness and stomach pains. These symptoms can be quite vague but still quite troublesome and these can often be relieved by following a gluten free diet.

Other reasons to avoid gluten would be if you suffered with a wheat allergy, and this is different from being a Coeliac. This is not an auto-immune condition, but a reaction to wheat, where swelling, itching, a rash and even anaphylactic shock could occur. As with any allergy, you can have a mild or adverse reaction.

There are some claims that gluten can cause weight gain and it may be possible to lose weight when following a gluten free diet, however these suggestions do not have any real medical evidence to back this up. It is worth thinking about the fact that if we were to avoid gluten, we may lose a little weight due to the ingredients that you won't be eating alongside them. For example, the butter on the bread, the cream and cheese in the pasta or the packet of crisps cooked in oil, containing gluten. You may also find you eat slightly less as gluten-free options aren't so readily available, requiring you to think a little more about the food you eat. The weight loss may just be accidental or coincidental.

It is important to remember, that gluten-free isn't necessarily healthy, with such great substitute flours available nowadays, there are a wealth of gluten free donuts, brownies, pies and puddings out there to be enjoyed, but still in moderation!

## *Where is Gluten Found?*

If you are on a strict Gluten-Free diet you will need to know where gluten hides when you are out and about as it isn't always obvious. Bread products and pasta tend to be quite straight forward and easy to spot, but how about the gluten lurking in other places? It can be found in beer, sauces, stews, cereals, food colourings, dressings, crisp "coating" on foods, oats, rye, malt and soup. When buying pre-made and processed foods and drinks and when eating out, it is important that you check food labels and ask the chef.

Other items that may contain gluten which could surprise you are, lip gloss, lip balm, herbal supplements, meat substitutes (seitan), cheesecake filling, sweets and chocolate bars, stamps and envelopes and play dough!

## *What Does Gluten DO?*

When you are a Coeliac, gluten will cause the lining of the small intestine to break down and make it more difficult for the body to absorb essential vitamins and minerals. It can bring about a number of other auto-immune diseases, such as Diabetes Type 1, multiple sclerosis, osteoporosis, neurological disorders, migraines and some cancers so it is vital to follow a gluten free diet correctly.

Further studies more recent, are indicating that gluten is classed as a "lectin" and we are ALL at risk to suffering from symptoms when this is consumed. A mild breakdown of the small intestine lining can lead to a condition called leaky gut and this can be the cause of a number of symptoms. It is believed that when the body experiences this leaky gut, it begins to attack the harmful bacteria in the body and it can also begin to attack its own healthy cells. This can lead to weight gain, bloating, abdominal discomfort, IBS, chronic fatigue and even rheumatoid arthritis.

There is on-going research into the problems some of us can encounter with gluten but the most sensible thing to do is to visit your health care provider if you feel you may have unexplained symptoms before embarking on any diet.

## *What Can I Eat?*

With gluten-free living on the increase worldwide, there is an incredibly easy and interesting array of grains and alternative foods to choose from. A culinary adventure of ingredients with different flavours, textures, vitamins and minerals from different sources, can only fill our bodies with good things.

Here is a list of all the gluten free grains* you can experiment with when making snacks. It is worth noting that the best results in gluten-free baking is when you combine different grains together and after a few attempts you should get some great fool proof results.

- Rice Flour
- Bean Flours (like chickpea flour)
- Cornmeal
- Buckwheat Flour
- Sorghum Flour
- Quinoa Flour
- Amaranth Flour

- Millet Flour
- Oat Flour
- Teff Flour
- Chestnut, Almond, Coconut and other Nut Flours
- Sweet Rice Flour
- Potato Flour
- Potato Starch
- Tapioca Flour/Starch (Cassava)
- Cornflour
- Arrowroot Flour
- Xanthan or Guar Gum (for combining baking ingredients in the absence of gluten)

*Make sure these flours are all certified Gluten Free as some are milled in factories making gluten flour.

## *Extra Tips for Gluten Free Cooking*

When you bake with gluten flours, they provide the binding properties needed to create soft bakes that rise, with the structured textures that we are used to. Experiment with different ingredients to try and add that softness to bakes. Flaxseed and soaked chia seeds are great binding agents.

Add cottage cheese or cream cheese to batters and snack mixes to make them softer.

Apple sauce (unsweetened) is a great gluten-free baker's friend and can add a welcome softness to a bake.

When making bakes that are sweet and you have found the results a little crumbly, add a vanilla sugar syrup to the top when it's warm (even piercing the top with a skewer to help absorb more), and the texture will be much softer.

If you make a mistake with your snack baking, don't throw it away! Can it be rescued? For example, if it has been too crumbly to stick together, could this be processed further to make breadcrumbs?

Sweet ones can make a great crumble top and savoury ones can make a great gratin topping or a coating for chips.

The different flavours and textures of gluten free bakes can be enhanced by adding dried fruits, zests and nuts to them.

Watch out if you share a kitchen with others who consume gluten in their diet. It is very easy to cross contaminate and some coeliacs in particular can have adverse reactions to even the tiniest amount of gluten.

## *Celebrate the foods you can eat...*

Whether you are gluten-free living or not, this collection of recipes will inspire you to widen your own repertoire of foods you consume. When we eat a variety of ingredients from different sources, we improve our nutrition and wellbeing and keep our gut healthy.

Put on your favourite apron and get ready to enjoy the gluten-free snack foods you can actually eat!

# The Recipes

## *Sweet Snacks*

Even though there are some great store brought gluten-free products emerging out there, it is certainly better to be able to produce your own. Not only is it more cost effective (gluten-free bakes seem to come with a bigger price tag!), you know exactly what goes into the food you are consuming.

We should all aim for less processed foods and even if you have a sweet tooth when following a gluten-free diet, there are still some quick sweet snacks you can put together. All these recipes could be eaten by non-gluten-free individuals so there really is no need to be making different recipes for everyone.

## Jam Popovers

Makes: 10

These popovers are so quick to make and use a lovely mix of flours for the pastry. You could use whatever jam flavour you want for this and even use a chocolate spread if you're feeling a little indulgent.

### **Ingredients**

- 2 tbsp brown rice flour
- 2 tbsp sorghum flour
- 2 tbsp tapioca flour
- 3 tbsp potato starch
- 4 tsp sugar
- 1 tbsp xanthan gum
- 1 egg, beaten
- 1 cup of cubed butter
- 2-3 tbsp cold water to mix

- 4 tbsp Raspberry Jam
- A little milk to brush

## **Instructions**

1. Mix the flours, starch, sugar, xanthan gum together in a bowl.
2. Add the cubed butter and rub in, until it resembles breadcrumbs.
3. Pour in the beaten egg and enough water to create a stiff dough. Leave to rest for 1 hour in the fridge.
4. Pre-heat the oven to 400°F/200°C/Gas Mark 6 and grease or line a baking tray.
5. Roll out the dough between two sheets of cling film, until ¼" thick. Get a large cookie cutter and cut out 8-10 circles (depending on your cutter) and place on the baking tray.
6. Place a spoonful of jam on one side of the circle and brush a little milk on the outer edge of the other side. Fold over the jam filling and using a fork, seal the one side to create a semi-circle with pretty fork indents. Continue with all of the pastry circles.
7. Place in the oven for 20-25 minutes until crisp and golden.

# Chunky Monkeys

Makes 12

These chunky cookies are healthy and delicious, with soft banana, crunchy pecans and studs of dark chocolate you won't be keeping these for long. Gluten-free biscuits can be one of the easiest bakes to get right first so if you are trying gluten-free for the first time, this one is the perfect start!

Make sure you use really ripe bananas as there is no added sugar in this recipe and sweetness only comes from the bananas and dark chocolate.

## **Ingredients**

- 1 ¼ cup of rolled oats
- ¼ cup of oat flour
- ½ tsp baking powder
- 2 ripe bananas
- 1 egg, beaten

- 2 tbsp pecans, chopped
- 2 tbsp dark chocolate chips (try to use 70% cocoa chocolate)

## Instructions:

1. Pre-heat the oven to 400°F/200°C/Gas Mark 6 and grease or line a baking tray.
2. Peel the bananas and mash in a bowl.
3. Add the rolled oats, oat flour, baking powder, pecans, dark chocolate and beaten egg and mix well to make sure the dough is well combined.
4. Place 12 mounds of the mix on the baking tray and bake for 15-20 minutes until the tops are golden and the cookies are cooked.
5. Cool on a wire rack and keep in an air tight container for 4-5 days (if they last that long!).

## Fruit Bakes

Makes: 12 bars

When cooking without gluten, it's really worth looking for recipes or adapting others with fruit purees, like apple sauce, pureed mango or mashed bananas. These can add the softness you can sometimes lose in gluten free baking, as it has a bit of a reputation to be a little crumbly.

These bakes are lovely as a snack, but they could also be added to a dessert plate with a dollop of cream, ice cream or even custard (gluten free of course)

### **Ingredients:**

- 4 tbsp maple syrup
- 1/3 cup of dairy free spread / butter, softened
- 1 large egg, beaten
- 1 ½ cups of apple sauce
- 1 ½ cups of gluten-free flour blend

- 2 tsp ground cinnamon
- 1 tsp baking powder
- Pinch of salt
- ½ cup of hazelnuts, chopped

**Instructions:**

1. Pre-heat the oven to 400°F/200°C/Gas Mark 6 and grease or line a small baking tray.
2. Place the softened butter, maple syrup, beaten egg and apple sauce into a bowl and beat well together.
3. Add the gluten-free flour blend, ground cinnamon, baking powder, salt and hazelnuts to the bowl and mix well.
4. Tip into the prepared tin and bake for 20-25 minutes until golden and little puffed up.
5. Allow to cool in the tin and then turn out onto a chopping board. Cut in to 12 slices and store in the fridge for 5-7 days in an air tight container.

# Chocolate Bean Cake

Serves: 8-10

Snacks should be quick and easy to put together and you wouldn't normally consider a cake to be a "quick and easy" option. However, if you have a food processor, this one takes minutes to put together and then it's just 25 minutes in the oven. You can use whatever tinned beans you have for this recipe, they add useful binding properties to gluten-free baking and also add some filling and energy giving protein.

## **Ingredients:**

- 3 tbsp olive oil
- 1 x 14oz red kidney beans (or other tinned beans would work)
- 1/3 cup of rice flour
- 3 tbsp cocoa powder
- 1 ½ tsp baking powder
- Pinch of salt

- 1 tsp vanilla extract
- 3 eggs
- ½ cup of light brown sugar

**Instructions:**

1. Pre-heat the oven to 400°F/200°C/Gas Mark 6 and grease or line an 8" round cake tin.
2. Place all of the ingredients into a food processor and blend. You may need to stop once or twice to scrape down the side.
3. Tip the mix in to the tin and bake for 25 minutes, until risen and a skewer comes out clean.
4. Cool in the pan for 10 minutes and then turn out and slice into wedges.
5. You could also make this into a dessert by adding a dollop of vanilla ice cream, cream or even a homemade custard.

# Citrus, Sultana and Polenta Slice

Serves: 10

These sultanas in this slice are soaked in the orange juice and this makes them so plump and juicy! Don't miss out this stage as it really makes a difference to the result. It may seem odd boiling the fruit beforehand but go with it as it creates a lovely soft texture without resorting to gluten.

## Ingredients:

- 2 lemons
- 2 oranges
- 2 tbsp orange juice
- ¾ cup of sultanas
- 1/3 cup of fine cornmeal (polenta, not quick cook)
- 1/3 cup of almond flour
- 2 tsp baking powder
- 4 eggs, beaten

- 1/3 cup of sugar

## Instructions:

1. Heat a saucepan of water up and add the lemons and oranges. Bring to a boil and simmer for an hour, until they are soft.
2. Place the sultanas in the orange juice and leave to soak.
3. Pre-heat the oven to 400°F/200°C/Gas Mark 6 and grease an 8"x8" square cake tin.
4. Slice the fruit up to remove the pips and the little stalks at the top.
5. Place all of the ingredients (leave out the sultanas), including the skin and everything else of the orange and lemon into a food processor. Blend until you have a really smooth batter.
6. Stir in the sultanas and pour into the prepared cake tin.
7. Bake for 30-35 minutes until risen and golden on top.
8. Cut in to slices to snack on.

# Chestnut and Apricot Jam Muffins

Makes: 10

Chestnut flour is a great ingredient for gluten free diets. It contains essential amino acids, dietary fiber and is also low in fat. It also provides vitamin E, Bs, potassium and magnesium so certainly worth adding to your snack repertoire.

## **Ingredients:**

- 1/3 cup of chestnut flour
- Pinch of salt
- 2 tsp baking powder
- 4 tbsp apricot jam
- 2 eggs, beaten
- 4 tbsp runny honey
- ½ tsp vanilla extract
- 4 tbsp olive oil
- 3 tbsp flaked almonds to finish

## **Instructions**

1. Pre-heat the oven to 400°F/200°C/Gas Mark 6 and place 10 paper cases in a muffin tin.

2. Heat the jam slightly to loosen it and leave it to one side.

3. Beat the eggs, oil, honey and vanilla together.

4. Place all of the Ingredients into a bowl and combine well.

5. Divide the mix between the paper cases and sprinkle over the flaked almonds

6. Bake for 20-25 minutes until risen and golden on top.

# Gluten-Free Biscotti

Makes: Approximately 18-20

This crunchy biscuit is the perfect snack to dunk in a cup of strong coffee. Biscotti means "double baked" and this does take a bit of effort. However, once made, these slices keep in an airtight container for a week and they are worth that double bake!

### **Ingredients:**

- 1 cup of gluten-free flour blend
- 2 tsp baking powder
- Pinch of salt
- ¾ cup of white sugar
- 1 ¼ cups of whole blanched almonds, chopped a little
- 4 eggs, beaten
- 2 tsp vanilla extract
- 1 tsp almond extract (optional)

## Instructions:

1. Pre-heat the oven to 375°F/190°C/Gas Mark 5 and line or grease a baking tray.

2. Add all of the ingredients into a bowl and beat well together. The mix will be quite wet.

3. Shape two log shapes of the dough alongside each other on the baking tray.

4. Bake for 20-25 minutes until lightly cooked, risen and a little coloured.

5. Leave to cool.

6. With a sharp, serrated knife, place the loaves on a chopping board and slice each in to 1 ½" thick pieces.

7. Place each slice back on to the baking tray.

8. Reduce the temperature of the oven to 300°F/150°C/Gas Mark 2.

9. Place the baking tray back in the oven for a further 25-30 minutes. The biscotti should be crisp and lightly coloured evenly all over, if not, return to the oven for a further 5-10 minutes.

10. Store in an airtight container for 7 days.

You could change the flavours of this if you like. Omit the almonds and almond essence and add hazelnut and chocolate chips. Or you could add chopped dried figs and chopped walnuts.

# Chestnut Flour and Brown Sugar Shortbread Wedges

Makes: 8-10

These snappy wedges are crisp and sweet. The brown sugar and vanilla adds a lovely caramel flavour and you could substitute the oil for 4oz of real butter. This would create a much creamier flavour than the olive oil, but should may be saved for special occasions if you are watching your saturated fat levels.

## **Ingredients:**

- 1/3 cup of chestnut flour
- 1/3 cip of ground almonds
- 1/3 cup of buckwheat flour
- Pinch of salt
- 1 tsp baking powder
- ¼ cup of light brown sugar
- 1/3 cup of Olive Oil

- 1 tsp vanilla extract

**Instructions:**

1. Pre-heat the oven to 400°F/200°C/Gas Mark 6 and grease or line a baking tray.
2. Mix all of the flours together and stir in the salt, baking powder and sugar.
3. Add the olive oil and mix together until it starts to clump together. Add a little iced cold water to help if it's too dry to form a dough. Place in the fridge for 20 minutes to rest.
4. Roll out the dough into a rough circle, about 1" thick and place on the baking tray. Mark partially through the dough to create 8-10 wedges.
5. Bake for 20-25 minutes until golden and crisp and then cut fully through the wedge markings.

## Peanut Oaties

Makes: 10-12

These oaties are full of great texture and flavour. You could add almond butter here instead of the peanuts and use chopped almonds instead of the raisins.

### Ingredients:

- ½ cup of crunchy peanut butter, no sugar added
- 3 tbsp runny honey
- 1 egg
- ¼ tsp baking soda
- ¼ cup of raisins
- 1/3 cup of rolled oats

## Instructions:

1. Pre-heat the oven to 400°F/200°C/Gas Mark 6 and grease or line a baking tray.

2. Mix all of the ingredients together until well combined.

3. Using a spoon, place mounds of the mix on to the baking tray and press down a little to make similar sized and shaped bites.

4. Bake for 15-20 minutes until cooked and golden.

# Ginger Cookies

Makes: 12-14

Ginger cookies are a firm favourite with families and this one uses the stem ginger in syrup. You can use the ginger for other recipes in this book too, so don't let it go to waste. The only other sweetener for them is in the dates, so they are quite healthy too with no refined sugars.

## **Ingredients:**

- 8 pitted dates, chopped
- 1 tbsp stem ginger syrup from a jar
- 1 ball of stem ginger, sliced finely
- ¾ cup of ground almonds
- ¼ cup of rice flour
- ¼ tsp baking soda
- 2 medium eggs

**Instructions:**

1. Pre-heat the oven to 400°F/200°C/Gas Mark 6 and grease or line a baking tray

2. Place the dates and ginger syrup into a mini food processor and blend until a smooth paste is formed.

3. Mix the paste with all of the other ingredients to form a dough. If it is a little dry, add a drop or two of milk (gluten free flours can be a little inconsistent with absorbency).

4. Add dollops of the cookie mix on to the baking tray and press down with a wet fork to make a little thinner.

5. Bake in the oven for 20-25 minutes until coloured and crisp.

# No Cook Rice Cake Bonanza!

All to Serve: 1

Sometimes you need a snack without the hassle of having to cook something. Assembly cooking in the kitchen is great for snacks as it takes minimal times, which is important when hunger is lurking!

You could use any number of neutral tasting, gluten-free crackers or biscuits for these toppings.

## *The Banana One*

### **Ingredients:**

- 2 large rice cakes
- 1 banans, peeled and mashed
- 1 tsp maple syrup
- 2 tbsp chopped pecans

**Instructions:**

1. Place the rice cakes on a plate.
2. Mash the banana with the honey and spread over the rice cakes.
3. Scatter over the pecans and enjoy.

## *The Nutty One*

**Ingredients:**

- 2 large rice cakes
- 2 tbsp peanut butter (no added sugar)
- 1 tsp honey
- ½ apple, sliced

**Instructions:**

1. Place the rice cakes on a plate.

2. Mash the butter and honey together and spread over the rice cakes.

3. Top with the slices of apples.

## The Apple One

### **Ingredients:**

- 2 large rice cakes
- 2 tbsp almond butter
- 2 tbsp apple sauce
- ½ tsp ground cinnamon
- 2 tbsp flaked almonds

### **Instructions:**

1. Place the rice cakes on a plate.
2. Spread on the almond butter.
3. Mix the apple sauce with the cinnamon and spread on top of the butter.

4. Scatter over the flaked almonds.

## The Chocolate One

### Ingredients:

- 2 large rice cakes
- 2 tbsp chocolate hazelnut spread
- ½ large banana, sliced
- 1 tbsp chopped roasted hazelnuts

### Instructions:

1. Place the rice cakes on a plate.
2. Spread the hazelnut spread on top.
3. Place the banana slices over the chocolate spread and then scatter over the hazelnuts

## *The Raspberry One*

### Ingredients:

- 2 large rice cakes
- 2 tbsp seedless raspberry jam (reduced sugar if you can find it)
- 2 tbsp cream cheese
- 2 tbsp black sesame seeds

### Instructions:

1. Place the rice cakes on a plate.
2. Spread the jam over the rice cakes and carefully spread the cream cheese on, without mixing too much.
3. Scatter over the sesame seeds.

## The S'mores One

### Ingredients:

- 2 large rice cakes
- 2 marshmallows
- 2 tbsp chocolate spread

### Instructions:

1. Place the rice cakes on a tray to go under a grill.
2. Spread the chocolate spread over.
3. Top with the marshmallows and toast briefly under the grill until crusty and coloured.
4. Allow to cool a little before consuming.

# Gluten-Free Funnel Cakes

Makes 8-10

This comforting snack is a bit like a string of donut, dusted in cinnamon and sugar. Make sure the ingredients are all gluten-free certified. Best enjoyed warm, freshly cooked.

### **Ingredients**:

- 1 cup of rice flour
- ½ cup of tapioca starch
- 2 tbsp sugar
- 1 tsp baking powder
- 1 tsp salt
- ¼ tsp xanthan gum
- 1 cup of milk
- 2 large eggs
- 2 tbsp fine white sugar and 1 tsp ground cinnamon to dust

- Vegetable oil to deep fry

**Instructions:**

1. Heat the oil to 375°F/200°C.

2. Whisk the rice flour, tapioca starch, baking powder, salt, xanthan gum, 2 tablespoons of sugar, milk and eggs together. Beat well until you have a smooth batter.

3. Pour the batter into a large freezer or food bag (this is done quite easily by placing the bag in a large glass and opening it up around and over the edges of the glass and pouring the batter in)

4. Carefully snip a small corner off the bottom of the bag, holding on to the hole. Let go and allow the batter to pour into the hot oil. Makes sure you draw a "scribble" of the batter that crosses over itself to create a lattice type pattern, about 5"-6" in diameter.

5. Cook for 2-3 minutes and then flip over and cook for a further 2-3 minutes until golden and cooked.

6. Meanwhile, mix the ground cinnamon and fine sugar on a plate.

7. Drain the cooked funnel cakes on kitchen towel and repeat until all of the batter is used up.

8. Whilst warm, dust in the sugar and cinnamon mix. Serve immediately.

# Brownies Gone Blonde

Makes: 9

Okay, this isn't really a healthy snack to be cooked up regularly, but as a weekend treat these blondies are a lovely snack to offer family and friends. This recipe uses an already blended gluten-free flour and there are some great products out there nowadays! Choose your favourite that has given you the best results or you could make your own blend up using a mix of the gluten-free grains listed on the introduction.

## **Ingredients:**

- 1 ½ sticks of melted butter
- 2 large eggs, beaten
- 1 tsp vanilla extract
- 1 ¼ cups of dark brown sugar
- 1 ½ cups of gluten-free flour (ready-made blend)
- 1 tsp baking powder (gluten-free)
- ½ tsp salt

- 1 cup of white chocolate chips

**Instructions:**

1. Pre-heat the oven to 400°F/200°C/Gas Mark 6 and line a baking tray, measuring approximately 8" x 8" square.

2. Beat the melted butter, eggs and vanilla extract together. Add the dark brown sugar and beat well until the sugar is dissolving and the mix is quite smooth.

3. Add the flour, baking powder, salt and white chocolate chips and mix until well combined.

4. Pour into the prepared tin and bake for 20 minutes or until shrinking away from the side and a little coloured. Don't overcook this as this blondie is best slightly under cooked, soft and very squidgy.

# Popped Corn!

Serves 4

Popcorn is a great treat for any gluten-free snack. You could make it as healthy, or unhealthy as you like. Here are some combinations you could do that will hopefully please any family.

## **Ingredients:**

- 1 cup of popcorn maize
- 1 tbps olive oil

Either use a popcorn maker (don't use the oil if so) or cook the corn in batches in a large saucepan. Heat the oil first, add a little corn and replace the lid. Wait until the "popping" stops before removing the popped corn and carrying on with the next batch.

When just warm still, add these flavours:

## Salted Caramel

- 4 tbsp butter
- 3 tbsp brown sugar
- 1 tsp sea salt flakes

Melt the ingredients together until smooth and caramel like. Allow to cool a little before adding to the popcorn as it will cause it to shrink.

## Mint Chocolate

- 6-8oz dark chocolate
- 5 leaves of mint, chopped finely

Melt the chocolate in a glass bowl over a pan of simmering water. Stir in the mint leaves.

Leave to cool down and then stir through the fresh popcorn.

## Cinnamon and Spice

- 4 tbsp butter
- 3 tbsp brown sugar
- 1 tsp ground cinnamon
- ½ tsp ground nutmeg

## Instructions:

1. In a saucepan add the butter and brown sugar until melted. Stir through the spices. Leave to cool a little.
2. Drizzle over the freshly popped popcorn.

# Ginger and Dark Chocolate Flapjack Cookies

Makes: 15

If you can, try to use chocolate with at least 70% cocoa for this recipe, the dark chocolate combines so well with the ginger and it isn't quite the same with the milk chocolate varieties.

Use the stem ginger in syrup from other recipes in this book as it's a great ingredient to use in baking, so it's worth getting and not wasting it!

## Ingredients:

- ½ cup of dark chocolate chips (at least 70% cocoa)
- ½ cup of dark brown sugar
- 1 ½ cup rolled oats
- 1 tsp baking soda
- 1 cup of rice flour
- 1 egg, beaten

- ½ cup dairy butter/spread
- 1 ball of stem ginger, shredded

**Instructions:**

1. Pre-heat the oven to 400°F/200°C/Gas Mark 6 and grease or line a baking tray.
2. Put the butter/spread in a saucepan with the sugar and stir over a medium heat, until melted.
3. Remove from the heat and then stir in the rolled oats, baking soda, rice flour, chocolate chips and stem ginger.
4. Shape in to 15 balls and flatten down on the baking tray.
5. Bake for 20-25 minutes, until golden and cooked.
6. Cool on a rack and store in an airtight container for 5-7 days.

# Gluten Free Snack Bread

Makes: 1 loaf

This wouldn't be a gluten-free snack book without a loaf of bread for you to use! This recipe produces a soft textured bread that could be used for a number of snacks. Make sure all of the flours and powders you use are certified gluten free.

Try some of the following snack recipes (and some more in the Savoury Chapter) to use the bread and wonder why living gluten-free could ever be a problem.

## Ingredients:

- ¾ cup of warm water
- 1 pack of instant yeast (7oz sachet)
- 1 ½ cups of millet flour
- 1 cup of tapioca starch
- 2 tbsp sugar

- 2 tsp xanthan gum

- 1 tsp salt

- ½ tsp baking powder (gluten-free)

- 3 eggs, beaten

- 2 tbsp olive oil

- 1 tsp apple cider vinegar

**Instructions:**

1. Mix the water and yeast together and allow to stand for 5 minutes,

2. Add the millet flour, tapioca starch, sugar, xanthan gum, salt and baking powder to a stand mixer bowl. Using the normal flat paddle attachment, mix the dry ingredient together.

3. Increase the speed and add the yeast mix, eggs, oil and vinegar. Mix until smooth.

4. Grease or line a small loaf tin and spread the dough inside.

5. Cover the tin with loose plastic wrap and leave in a warm place for about one hour.

6. When the dough has doubled in size, pre-heat the oven to 350°F/180°C/Gas Mark 4 and remove the wrap.

7. Bake the bread for 40-45 minutes. If the top is getting a bit too coloured before it is cooked, place some aluminium foil on top to protect the crust.

8. Remove the bread from the oven and allow to cool for a few minutes before removing from the tin.

9. Cool completely before slicing as it will be quite difficult to cut warm.

## French Toasties (using the gluten-free snack loaf)

Serves: 2

When you have a good loaf of gluten-free bread there really is no reason to be avoiding comfort foods like this eggy snack. Perfect for a snack before bedtime with its calming cinnamon and the sleep inducing tryptophan from the eggs.

**Ingredients:**

- 4 small slices of gluten-free bread
- 2 eggs, beaten
- 2 tbsp milk
- 1 tbsp fine white sugar
- 1 tsp ground cinnamon
- 1 tbsp olive oil

**Instructions:**

1. Heat a frying pan and add the oil.
2. Mix the egg and milk together until well combined.
3. Dip the bread pieces in the egg and milk mix, making sure they absorb all of the liquid evenly.
4. Gently lay the bread pieces in the hot oil and cook over a medium heat until golden.
5. Meanwhile, spread the sugar and ground cinnamon on a plate and mix well to combine.

6. When the bread is cooked, remove from the pan and lay straight into the sugar mix. Make sure both sides are gently coated.

7. Serve immediately.

# Fruit Topped Bread (using the gluten-free snack loaf)

Serves 1

When you have bread that tastes this good, you don't have to do much to it. This recipe uses some ripe, sweet strawberries which have bucket loads of vitamin C. The cream cheese is a great source of calcium and you could easily change this to the lower fat versions if you are on a weight loss goal.

The scattering of seeds on top adds a lovely crunchy texture and nutty flavour.

## **Ingredients:**

- 1 thick wedge of gluten-free snack bread
- 2 tbsp cream cheese
- 6 strawberries
- 1 tbsp pumpkin seeds

**Instructions:**

1. Spread the cream cheese on to the bread.

2. Hull the strawberries and thinly slice them.

3. Arrange the strawberry slices over the cream cheese and bread.

4. Scatter the pumpkin seeds over the top and enjoy this summery, filling snack any time.

# Baked Banana and Chocolate Fingers (using the gluten-free snack loaf)

Serves 1

This one is a great, simple snack for children and should maybe be saved for a treat for when they have arranged a play date.

Served with a glass of milk, it could also be a lovely bed time snack for all ages.

## Ingredients:

- 2 slices of the gluten-free snack bread
- 1 small banana, peeled and sliced
- 1 tbsp chocolate and hazelnut spread

**Instructions:**

1. Pre-heat the oven to 400°F/200°C/Gas Mark 6 and line a baking tray with foil.

2. Lie the snack bread out on a board. Spread the chocolate spread on to one side.

3. Evenly place the banana slices on top of the chocolate spread and then top with the other slice of bread.

4. Place on the baking tray and bake for 7-8 minutes until toasty and the banana oozing.

5. Serve with a napkin!

## Fruity Kebabs

Serves 2

This snack is put together using ready-made gluten-free scone pieces. You could use the following recipe if you wanted to try making them yourself as they are really easy and taste great.

You could pack these for children in their lunch boxes, but it may be better to use a plastic drinking straw instead of a metal and wooden skewer. Use different fruits but add lots of colour!

**<u>Ingredients</u>**:

- 6 strawberries, small
- 1 peach
- 6 red grapes
- 2 kiwis
- 1 gluten-free scone

**Instructions:**

1. Hull the strawberries and thread the strawberries on to the skewers/straws.

2. Slice the peach in half, twist and remove the stone. Cut in to 4 chunks. Thread on to the skewers too.

3. Thread the grapes on.

4. Peel the kiwis and cut both in to 4 chunks each. Thread on to the skewers

5. Cut the scones in to 2 pieces and thread last on to the skewers.

You could dip these into yoghurt, drizzle over some maple syrup or just enjoy as they are.

# Fruit Scones

Makes 9

Scones are a tea time favourite and can be actually be made quite healthy if you are on a weight loss goal. You don't have to serve them with lashings of clotted cream and fruit jam, but you could create your own sugar free fruit spread (like this one) and serve with a refreshing dollop of Greek yoghurt.

## **Ingredients:**

- 1 cup of gluten-free flour
- ½ cup of oat flour (gluten free)
- 2 tsp baking powder (gluten free)
- ¼ cup of almond flour
- A pinch of salt
- 5 tbsp of dairy free spread/butter
- 3 tbsp raisins or sultanas (optional)
- 3-4 tbsp milk

## Instructions:

1. Pre-heat the oven to 400°F/200°C/Gas Mark 6 and grease or line a baking tray.

2. Place the gluten-free flour, oat flour, baking powder, almond flour, salt and the dairy free spread or butter into a bowl. Using a knife, cut the butter in to the dry ingredients to form a coarse mix that resembles bread crumbs.

3. Add enough milk to create a firm dough.

4. Place the dough between two sheets of cling film and roll out to a thickness of about 1".

5. Cut 9 rounds of the dough out, using a cookie cutter and place on the baking tray.

6. Place in the oven and bake for 15-20 minutes until risen and golden.

7. Remove from the oven and place on a wire rack to cool.

## For the Fruit Spread

This recipe can be used for many snack ideas. How about simply spreading on to gluten-free bread with some butter? Top a rice pudding with it? Just eat with yoghurt or add to a smoothie?

The chia seeds add the jelly like consistency you find in jams and the only sweetener is a little maple syrup, but if you are using ripe and sweet berries you could even leave this out.

### Ingredients:

- 1 cup of strawberries (you can use any other berries you like)
- 1 tbsp maple syrup (optional)
- 2 tbsp water
- 2 tbsp chia seeds

**Instructions:**

1. Chop the strawberries up until quite fine, you still want a little texture though. Mix with the water and the chia seeds and place in the fridge in a jar for 3 hours at least.

2. This can be stored in the fridge for up to 1 week.

# Mug Cake Snacks

A mug cake is a wonderful snack to fill a gap. They take minutes to prepare and cook and can be healthy or unhealthy! These two recipes give you the best of both worlds so pick the one that fits with your eating objectives. Sometimes an indulgent treat is good for the soul, but you don't need to step off the diet to enjoy the healthier version!

## *Chocolate Chip Mug Cake (indulgent)*

Serves 1

### **Ingredients**

- 3 tbsp oat flour or gluten-free flour blend
- 2 tbsp of light brown sugar
- Pinch of salt
- 2 tbsp melted butter
- 1 egg
- 2 tbsp milk

- 1 tsp vanilla extract

- 1 tbsp chocolate chips

- Ice cream to serve (optional)

## **Instructions:**

1. Place all of the ingredients into a bowl and beat until really smooth.

2. Find a microwaveable mug and tip the mixture in.

3. Place in the microwave and cook on "high" for 1-1 ½ minutes or until risen and cooked. Place a dollop of ice cream on top if you really need a treat!

## *Fudgy Chocolate Cake Mug (the healthier version)*

Serves 1

### **Ingredients**

- 2 tbsp cocoa powder
- 2 tbsp oat flour
- 2 tbsp maple syrup
- 1 egg
- 2 tbsp skimmed milk or almond milk
- ½ tbsp olive oil

### **Instructions**

1. Whisk the ingredients together in a bowl until smooth.
2. Pour into a microwaveable mug and cook on "high" for 1-1 ½ minutes, until risen and cooked. It is best to slightly undercook this as the mug cake will be more fudge-like and feel more luxurious.

# Oat Apple Balls

Makes 10

These bite size apple balls are a tasty snack to be popping into the mouth and they are super healthy too. No added sugars and all the benefits from a fresh apple grated into the mix. Try to find a red skinned apple as it creates a lovely pink fleck throughout and they can be extra sweet.

## **Ingredients**

- 2 dessert apples
- ¼ cup of walnuts, chopped
- 2 tbsp maple syrup
- 1 tsp ground cinnamon
- 1 cup of rolled oats
- ½ cup of almond flour
- ¼ cup of desiccated coconut
- 1 egg, beaten

- 1 tbsp flaxseed

## **Instructions**

1. Pre-heat the oven to 400°F/200°C/Gas Mark 6 and grease or line a baking tray.
2. Grate the apple, without peeling. Squeeze out any extra moisture and add to a bowl.
3. Place the chopped walnuts, maple syrup, rolled oats, almond flour, ground cinnamon, desiccated coconut, beaten egg and flaxseed into the bowl with the apple and mix to combine well.
4. Using a tablespoon (or damp hands), create approximately 10 balls of the mix and place on the baking tray.
5. Bake for 15-20 minutes until the balls are golden and crisp on the outside.
6. Store in an air tight container for 5-7 days.

## *Savoury Snacks*

There really is no need to miss out on the usual savoury snacks that you would normally enjoy when you're following a gluten-free diet. There are some great flour blends out there that can create quite similar textures to gluten flour and some even provide more nutrition and more taste.

For quick snacks, look out for the gluten-free crackers and wraps that you can transform quite easily into a tasty quick dish, with hardly no cooking required. There are some great topping and wrap filling ideas to get creative with in these following recipes.

## Flaxseed Wraps

Makes: 4 wraps

### **Ingredients**

- 1 ½ cup of fine flaxseed
- 1 cup of water
- ½ tsp salt
- ¼ tsp garlic powder
- ¼ ground ginger
- ¼ tsp onion powder
- ¼ tsp ground cumin

### **Instructions**

1. Pour the water in to a saucepan and bring to a boil.

2. Remove from the heat and place all of the ingredients into the water in one go. Stir immediately and keep stirring for 1-2 minutes.

3. The mix will start quite wet but then it will start sticking together and coming away from the sides of the saucepan in one ball.

4. Remove from the saucepan and place between two sheets of baking parchment.

5. Roll out until about ¼" and then remove the top layer of paper and then using a diner plate, cut out a round circle.

6. Heat a non-stick frying pan and add the circle of dough into the pan. Cook for 1-2 minutes on both sides until lightly coloured and cooked.

7. Remove and keep under a tea towel, to prevent drying out.

## *Here are some ideas to fill the wrap*

- A handful of prawns mixed with a little mayonnaise, chopped chives and lemon zest.
- ½ an avocado, stone removed and peeled and sliced, 1 tbsp pumpkin seeds, 1 slice of ham.

- ½ ball of mozzarella, sliced, 3-4 basil leaves, shredded, plum tomato, sliced.

- ½ small tin of tuna, 1 tbsp mayonnaise, 2 tbsp sweetcorn, 1 tbsp flat leaf parsley chopped.

- 2 eggs, scrambled, 2 spring onions, shredded, 1 tbsp nutritional yeast.

# Chinese Prawn Snack Rolls

Makes: 10

Rice papers are naturally gluten free and this recipe is good example of how you don't always have to try to make substitutes of your favourite dishes. You could just enjoy the traditional dishes and snacks that are already gluten free and celebrate the foods you CAN eat.

Feel free to change the vegetables you add to this dish and even the meat. You could replace the prawns with minced chicken or keep them vegetarian.

## **Ingredients**

- 10 rice paper wrappers
- 1 tsp olive oil
- 1 garlic clove, crushed
- 1 medium carrot, shredded
- 3 spring onions, shredded

- 2 chinese lettuce leaves, shredded
- 1 tbsp black sesame seeds
- ½ cup of cooked prawns, chopped
- ¼ tsp Chinese 5 spice powder
- 1 tsp toasted sesame seed oil
- ½ tsp salt
- Olive oil for brushing and extra sesame seeds for sprinkling

## **Instructions**

1. Pre-heat the oven to 400°F/200°C/Gas Mark 6 and grease or line a baking tray.
2. In a frying pan, heat the oil and add the spring onion, crushed garlic, carrot and lettuce leaves. Stir over a high heat to soften the ingredients.
3. Add the prawns and stir to heat through.
4. Add the sesame seeds, Chinese 5 spice powder, toasted sesame oil and salt and stir well.
5. Meanwhile, place the rice paper wrappers in a bowl of water to soften for 5 minutes. It is better to do this one at a

time as if they soak for too long they will break when you try to roll them up.

6. Place a spoonful of the mix on top of a softened rice paper wrapper and then fold over the edges. Roll up carefully to fully enclose the filling and place on the baking tray.

7. Repeat with all ten wrappers and then brush with the olive oil. Sprinkle over some extra sesame seeds and place in the oven for 10 minutes to crisp up.

8. Cool a little and serve with some chilli sauce for dipping.

# Muffin Mugs

Serves 2

These little mugs are quick and offer a lovely savoury gluten free snack for 2 hungry people. There are a number of flavours to try and they could be served at any time of the day.

## Cheese and Ham

### **Ingredients**

- 8 tbsp of oat flour or gluten-free flour blend
- 1 tsp baking powder
- ½ tsp salt
- 2 tbsp milk
- 2 eggs, beaten
- 2 tbsp olive oil
- 2 tbsp grated cheese
- 2 tbsp finely chopped ham

## **Instructions**

1. Beat the ingredients together well until combined.
2. Pour the mix into two greased mugs that can be used in the microwave.
3. Heat on "high" for 1- 1 ½ minutes until cooked and risen.
4. These should be eaten immediately after cooking.

## *Sour Cream and Onion*

## **Ingredients**

- 8 tbsp of oat flour or gluten-free flour blend
- 1 tsp baking powder
- 2 tbsp sour cream
- 4 spring onions, shredded
- 2 eggs, beaten
- 2 tbsp olive oil

## Instructions

1. Beat the ingredients together well until combined.
2. Pour the mix into two greased mugs that can be used in the microwave.
3. Heat on "high" for 1- 1 ½ minutes until cooked and risen.
4. These should be eaten immediately after cooking.

## Walnut and Feta

## Ingredients

- 8 tbsp of oat flour or gluten-free flour blend
- 1 tsp baking powder
- ½ tsp salt
- 2 tbsp milk
- 2 eggs, beaten
- 2 tbsp olive oil
- 2 tbsp chopped feta
- 2 tbsp chopped walnut

- ¼ tsp dried thyme

## **Instructions**

1. Beat the ingredients together well until combined.
2. Pour the mix into two greased mugs that can be used in the microwave.
3. Heat on "high" for 1- 1 ½ minutes until cooked and risen.
4. These should be eaten immediately after cooking.

# Courgette and Feta Cakes

Makes 8

These little cakes are best baked in the bottom of muffin tins to keep their shape whilst cooking. The feta adds a tasty saltiness to the flavour and also improves your calcium levels.

## **Ingredients**

- 1 cup of cooked quinoa
- 3 salad onions, shredded
- 1 egg, beaten
- ¼ cup feta, cubed
- 1 medium courgette, grated
- 1 tbsp nutritional yeast
- Small bunch of flat leaf parsley, chopped

**Instructions**

1. Pre-heat the oven to 400°F/200°C/Gas Mark 6 and grease a muffin tray.

2. Squeeze the courgettes to make sure as much moisture as possible is removed.

3. Mix all of the ingredients together and shape in the bottom of the muffin tin.

4. Place in the oven and bake for 25 minutes, until golden. Leave to cool in the tin before trying to remove.

# Socca with an Herb Crust

Makes 2 Flatbreads

This gluten free flatbread is make from chickpea flour and is a great snack to take out with you. You could leave the mix in the fridge for 48 hours and could even cook them fresh as and when they are needed as they taste great just out of the frying pan.

## **Ingredients**

- 1 cup of chickpea flour
- 1 tsp onion powder
- 1 tsp garlic powder
- ½ tsp salt
- 2 ¼ cups of water

## *Herb Topping*

- 2 tbsp chopped hazelnuts

- 2 tbsp sesame seeds

- 1 tsp ground cumin

- 1 tsp ground coriander

- 1 tbsp dried thyme

- ½ tbsp dried mint

- ½ tsp sea salt

- 2 tbsp olive oil to cook + extra for serving

**Instructions**

1. To make the topping, place the hazelnuts, sesame seeds, ground coriander, ground cumin, thyme, mint and salt into a pestle and mortar and give a good bash. You want it quite coarse still and with all the ingredients mixed well. Leave to one side.

2. To make the soccas, mix the chickpea flour together with the onion powder, garlic powder and salt. Add the water and whisk well until smooth. You should have a thick batter, add a little more water if not. Leave to one side for at least 1-2 hours.

3. When ready to cook, spoon off any froth from the top of the socca mix. Heat a large frying pan and add 1 tbsp of olive

oil. When really hot, pour half of the batter into the pan and cook over a medium heat for 4-5 minutes. Flip over and cook for a further 3-4 minutes, until crisp and golden. Remove the bread from the pan and place on a plate. Brush a little extra oil on the top of the socca (approximately 1 tbsp) whilst it is still warm and sprinkle 1 tbsp of the herb topping all over the top. Leave to cool. Repeat with the remaining batter.

4. Serve at room temperature either as it is, or with toppings of your choice or just a scattering of fresh herbs.

# Baked Garlic Mushroom Bites

Makes: 18

The coconut flour and ground almonds provide a great texture to these oven baked mushrooms. You could use a couple of slices of gluten-free bread and make them into breadcrumbs in a food processor, but this method is much easier and requires less washing up.

## **Ingredients**

- 18 medium chestnut mushrooms
- 2 tbsp arrowroot
- 2 egg whites, beaten together
- 2 tbsp coconut flour
- 2 tbsp ground almonds
- 1 tsp salt
- ½ tsp garlic powder
- 2 tbsp olive oil

## Instructions

1. Pre-heat the oven to 400°F/200°C/Gas Mark 6 and line a baking tray.

2. Pour the oil in to the tray and heat in the oven.

3. Dust the mushrooms in the arrowroot and then dip in the egg white.

4. Mix the coconut flour, ground almonds, salt and garlic powder on a plate and then dip the mushrooms in them, so they stick to the egg white.

5. When all the mushrooms have been coated, remove the tray from the oven and carefully place the mushrooms in the hot oil. Use a spoon to turn them over so they so they are covered in the oil.

6. Return the tray to the oven for 20 minutes and cook until the crisp.

7. Drain and eat immediately.

# Sesame Seed Crackers

Makes 60+ mini crackers

## **Ingredients**

- 3 cups of almond flour
- 1 tsp sea salt
- 1 tbsp rosemary leaves, chopped finely
- 1 cup of sesame seeds
- 2 eggs, beaten
- 2 tbsp olive oil

## **Instructions**

1. Pre-heat the oven to 350°C/180°C/Gas Mark 4 and get two sheets of parchment/baking paper out ready.
2. Mix all of the ingredients together until well combined.
3. Roll the dough between the two sheets of baking paper until really thin (about 1/8" thick).

4. Using a pizza cutter or knife, cut the dough into 2" squares and place on one of the sheets of baking paper.

5. Bake in the oven on a baking tray for 15 minutes until crisp and coloured.

## Parsnip and Rosemary Fries

Serves: 4 as a snack

Most people seem to love chips, and these are a great alternative. You could use potatoes or even sweet potatoes for this recipe too.

### **Ingredients**

- 6 parsnips, cut into batons
- 2 tbsp olive oil
- 3 tbsp fine cornmeal
- ½ tsp garlic powder
- ½ tsp sea salt
- 1 tbsp fresh rosemary, finely chopped

### **Instructions**

1. Pre-heat the oven to 400°C/200°C/Gas Mark 6 and grease or line a baking tray.

2. Add 1 tbsp of the oil to the baking tray and put in the oven to heat.

3. Dry the parsnips with kitchen towel.

4. Mix the cornmeal, garlic powder, salt and rosemary together on a plate.

5. Drizzle the other 1 tbsp of olive oil over the parsnips and then toss in the cornmeal mix on the plate.

6. Remove the tray from the oven and carefully place the parsnips on the tray, covering in the oil.

7. Return to the oven for 20 minutes until crisp and cooked.

# Mini Pizza Bites

Makes: 12

Pizza is extremely popular, but if you are living gluten-free, it unfortunately isn't really on the menu. However, that was before the introduction of some great gluten-free flours to make a great pizza base!

This dough used for these mini pizza bases is a wonderful recipe for a snack as it contains no yeast. This means you won't need to knead the dough and wait for it to prove. These bases can be ready in minutes and the most time spent will be finding the yummiest pizza toppings.

## **Ingredients (Dough)**

- 2 ½ cups of cassava flour
- 3 tsp baking powder (gluten free)
- 1 tsp salt
- 1 tsp sugar

- 1 tbsp olive oil
- 1 ¼ cups of water

## **Ingredients (Topping)**

- 2/3 cup of tomato sauce (homemade is best)
- 1 ball of mozzarella, roughly torn
- 8-10 leaves of fresh basil
- ½ cup of grated cheddar cheese
- 1 tsp dried oregano
- 1 tsp dried thyme

## **Instructions**

1. Pre-heat the oven to 400°F/200°C/Gas Mark 6 and grease or line a baking tray.
2. Place the cassava flour, baking powder, salt, sugar, olive oil and water in a bowl and mix well.
3. When combined, briefly knead it to create 12 small round pizza bases and place on the prepared baking tray.

4. Spoon a little of the tomato sauce on to each base, leaving a small margin clear around the edge. Add the mozzarella cheese between them.

5. Roughly tear the basil leaves and divide between the bases.

6. Sprinkle on the cheddar cheese and the dried herbs.

7. Place in the oven to bake for 15-20 minutes, or until the cheese is melted and golden on top.

8. Serve immediately or make up in advance to keep in the fridge for up to 5 days.

# Mozzarella Sticks

Makes 18-20

This recipe has been made a bit healthier by baking these stringy sticks instead of deep frying them, but feel free to cook them either way. These are great calcium filled snack that will certainly fill you up until the next meal.

## **Ingredients**

- 1 large block firm mozzarella, cut into sticks
- 1 egg
- 2 tbsp coconut flour
- 1 tbsp almond flour
- 1 tbsp buckwheat flour
- 1 tsp nutritional yeast
- 1 tsp garlic powder
- A little olive oil to drizzle over, a spray oil works well

**Instructions**

1. Beat the egg and place in a bowl.

2. Mix the coconut flour, almond flour, buckwheat flour, nutritional yeast and garlic powder together and place on a plate.

3. Dip each mozzarella stick into the beaten egg, drain and little and then coat in the flour mix.

4. Place on the tray.

5. Repeat until all of the cheese sticks have been used.

6. Place them in the fridge for 1-2 hours to allow to harden a little as this will make the cooked result much firmer.

7. Pre-heat the oven to 400°F/200°C/Gas Mark 6 and grease or line a baking tray.

8. Place all of the mozzarella sticks on to the baking tray and drizzle them all with a little oil to help them crisp up.

9. Bake for 10-15 minutes until the outside is golden and the middle is wanting to ooze out.

10. Eat immediately.

# Ricotta and Spinach Flatbread

Serves: 6-8

This flatbread is made from the pizza base recipe and shows how quickly a snack can be put together that's full of flavour.

Use a good quality extra-virgin olive oil for drizzling as it will really make a difference to the end result.

## **Ingredients**

- 2 ½ cups of cassava flour
- 3 tsp baking powder (gluten free)
- 1 tsp salt
- 1 tsp sugar
- 1 tbsp olive oil
- 1 ¼ cups of water
- 2/3 cup of ricotta
- 1 lemon, zest only

- 6-7 fresh basil leaves, shredded
- 1 ½ cup of fresh spinach leaves
- 1 tsp salt
- ¼ tsp nutmeg
- 1 garlic clove, crushed
- 2 tbsp of freshly grated parmesan cheese
- 1 tbsp dried oregano
- 1 tbsp of toasted pine nuts (optional)
- Extra-virgin olive oil to drizzle

## **Instructions**

1. Pre-heat the oven to 400°F/200°C/Gas Mark 6 and grease or line a baking tray.
2. Place the cassava flour, baking powder, salt, sugar, olive oil and water in a bowl and mix well.
3. When combined, briefly knead and create one large flatbread shape and place on the prepared baking tray.
4. Wash the spinach leaves and steam them in a saucepan with just the water on the leaves still. Give the leaves a

good squeeze to get the water out and stir in the nutmeg and salt. Roughly chop

5. Mix the ricotta with the garlic, salt and lemon zest and dollop over the flatbread. Do the same with the basil leaves and spinach and dried oregano.

6. Place in the oven for 15-20 minutes until the base is cooked and the golden.

7. Drizzle over a good helping of olive oil and the pine nuts (if using) before cutting in to 6-8 wedges.

# Green Crisps

Serves: 4

Sometimes you just need something crispy, savoury yet utterly healthy. These easy to create, gluten-free cabbage crisps are salty and moreish. Much better for you than the deep-fried bags of crisps, guaranteed to be without gluten and a great source of vitamin A, C, K, folate and calcium. Eating your greens has never tasted so good.

## **Ingredients**

- 3 cups of kale leaves, cavolo nero, curly cabbage (any hardy cabbage)
- 1 tbsp coconut oil, melted (or olive oil)
- 1 tsp sea salt

## Instructions

1. Pre-heat the oven to 400°F/200°C/Gas Mark 6 and grease or line a couple of baking trays.

2. Make sure the large fibrous stems have been removed from the cabbage leaves and cut in to large "crisp" size pieces.

3. Massage the oil and the salt into the leaves.

4. Tip on the baking trays and bake for 10-15 minutes until crisp and a little browned.

5. Eat immediately or these can be stored in an airtight container for 24 hours.

# Carrot Cornbread

Makes 9-10 pieces

This gluten free cornbread is made into a healthy snack with the addition of grated carrot. Carrot contains the plant compound, beta-carotene and provides the body with essential vitamin A and antioxidants.

## **Ingredients**

- 2 cups of fine cornmeal
- 2 tsp baking powder
- 1 tsp salt
- 2 eggs, beaten
- 1 1/3 cups of unsweetened almond milk
- 2 tbsp olive oil
- 2 cups of grated carrot

## Instructions

1. Pre-heat the oven to 375°C/190°C/Gas Mark 5 and grease an 8"x8" square baking tray.

2. Squeeze any moisture from the carrots and add to a bowl with the beaten egg, milk and olive oil and stir well.

3. In another bowl add the salt, cornmeal and baking powder and stir together.

4. Stir the carrot mix into the dry ingredients, combining well.

5. Pour the batter in to the baking tin and bake for 35-40 minutes until risen, coloured and cooked.

# Savoury Pan Scones

Makes: 15-20

These yummy little scones are so easy to make, and they store well too. Briefly re-heat them if you are in the kitchen, or they can be eaten from cold with a good quality salt crusted butter for a little treat.

## **Ingredients**

- 1 tbsp olive oil
- 1 cup of buckwheat flour
- ½ cup of rice flour
- ½ cup of cassava flour
- 1 tsp salt
- 2 tbsp dried oregano
- ½ tsp garlic powder
- 5 spring onions, shredded
- 3 tbsp parmesan cheese, grated

- 1 egg, beaten
- Approx 1 ¼ cups of unsweetened almond milk

## Instructions

1. Beat the eggs and milk together.
2. Stir the cheese, onions, garlic powder, oregano and flours together until well combined.
3. Beat in the egg mix until smooth. You need a thick milkshake consistency so add a little more or less milk to achieve this.
4. Heat the oil in a large frying pan and cook 3-4 spoons of the batter at once for 2-3 minutes on both sides.
5. Keep them warm until all of the batter is used up.
6. Enjoy immediately.

# Bacon Salad Cups

Makes: 4

Instead of messing about creating a carbohydrate to resemble something that is similar to gluten, how about bypassing that and just using a piece of bacon? Meat lovers would thank you for this savoury snack, regardless of whether they are following a gluten-free diet or not.

Romaine lettuce or rocket do tend to have the best nutrition when it comes to lettuces. The darker leaves give the most vitamins and is good rule to apply when choosing salad items.

This could be a great buffet dish to suit both gluten-free guests and gluten eating ones.

## **Ingredients**

- 8 slices of streaky bacon, unsmoked

- 1 cup of shredded salad leaves, romaine, rocket, baby gem, etc.
- 2 plum tomatoes, chopped, seeds removed
- 4 chunks of cucumber, seeds removed and finely chopped
- 4 mini balls (or pearls) of mozzarella

## **Instructions**

1. Preheat the oven to 400°F/200°C/Gas Mark 6 and grease 4 holes of a muffin tin.
2. Curl two slices of the bacon around the bottom and sides of the muffin holes, to create a "cup" shape.
3. Place the tray in the oven and bake for 15 minutes until the bacon is cooked, crisp and holding its shape. Allow to cool to room temperature.
4. Place the cups onto plates and fill with the salad leaves, chopped tomato and cucumber. Top with the mozzarella and enjoy.

# Cauliflower Wraps

Makes: 4-6

These wraps are easy to make; and they also perform really well as a sandwich filling vessel. They don't crack when rolled up and they will also count as one of your five a day! You could make a batch up and keep them in the fridge for 3-4 days so it's a good recipe to make for one person following a gluten-free diet.

## **Ingredients**

- ½ medium head of cauliflower
- 1 tsp onion powder
- ½ tsp garlic powder
- 2 tbsp cilantro, chopped
- 1 ½ cups of almond flour
- ¼ cup of psyllium husk
- 2 tbsp flaxseed
- 2 eggs, beaten

- ¼ cup oat flour
- A little olive oil to cook

## **Instructions**

1. Place the cauliflower in a blender and process until it resembles rice. It doesn't take long so watch it carefully as you don't want to end up with a very wet mix!

2. Mix the cauliflower with the powders, flours, psyllium husk, flaxseed, eggs and coriander and leave to thicken for 30 minutes.

3. Oil a large frying pan and roll out 4 rounds of dough. If it's still a little sticky you can push out with floured fingers and not use a rolling pin.

4. Cook each separately for 4-5 minutes on both sides, until golden and cooked.

5. Add any fillings that you like, or just enjoy warm straight from the pan.

## Cloud Bread Bakes

Makes: 6

This bread is a gluten-free, carbohydrate free snack that could be eaten anytime of the day. You could cook a batch and serve as part of a healthy breakfast buffet, accompanied by fresh fruits or just cook to enjoy as a tasty snack. They are better enjoyed straight from the oven when they are warm and puffed up.

### **Ingredients**

- 2 tbsp cream cheese
- 2 eggs, separated
- ¼ tsp baking powder (gluten free)

### **Instructions**

1. Pre-heat the oven to 300°F/150°C/Gas Mark 2 and grease a baking tray.

2. Place the egg whites in a bowl and whisk until they are stiff and won't tip out if tipped upside down.

3. Whisk together the cream cheese, egg yolks and baking powder until smooth and frothy.

4. Carefully fold the egg whites in, bit by bit. You don't want to lose much air from the egg whites so take your time with this step and use a large, metal spoon to make this easier.

5. Place 6 heaps of the mixture on to the baking tray.

6. Bake in the oven for 15-20 minutes until the bread is puffed up and golden.

7. Enjoy warm from the oven.

# Parmesan Funnel Cakes

Makes 8-10

These are a great social snack to make and it won't make any difference that the recipe uses gluten-free ingredients, so no need to tell! These are best eaten warm and you could use a different cheese if you would like.

## **Ingredients**

- 1 cup of rice flour
- ½ cup of tapioca starch
- 1 tsp baking powder
- 1 tsp salt
- ¼ tsp xanthan gum
- 1 cup of milk
- 2 large eggs
- 4 tbsp freshly grated parmesan
- Vegetable oil to deep fry

## Instructions

1. Heat the oil to 375°F/200°C.

2. Whisk the rice flour, tapioca starch, baking powder, salt, xanthan gum, 2 tablespoons of the cheese, milk and eggs together. Beat well until you have a smooth batter.

3. Pour the batter into a large freezer or food bag (this is done quite easily by placing the bag in a large glass and opening it up around and over the edges of the glass and pouring the batter in)

4. Careful snip a small corner off the bottom of the bag, holding on to the hole. Let go and allow the batter to pour into the hot oil. Makes sure you draw a "scribble" of the batter that crosses over itself to create a lattice type pattern, about 5"-6" in diameter.

5. Cook for 2-3 minutes and then flip over and cook for a further 2-3 minutes until golden and cooked.

6. Drain on kitchen towel and repeat until all of the batter is used up.

7. Whilst warm, sprinkle over the remaining parmesan cheese and serve.

# Coconut Spiced Funnel Cakes

Makes 8-10

These funnel cakes have a warming, spiced, curry flavour. Dotted with sesame seeds that provide some welcome protein, they bring a lovely nuttiness to the batter.

Using coconut milk here creates a soft and sweet batter that could be a great side dish for an Indian inspired meal or just enjoyed with an ice-cold beer in the garden with friends.

## **Ingredients**

- 1 cup of rice flour
- ½ cup of tapioca starch
- 1 tsp baking powder
- 1 tsp salt
- 1 tsp ground cumin
- ½ tsp ground turmeric

- 1 tsp garam masala
- 2 tbsp sesame seeds
- ¼ tsp xanthan gum
- 1 cup of coconut milk
- 2 large eggs
- 4 tbsp freshly grated parmesan
- Vegetable oil to deep fry

## **Instructions**

1. Heat the oil to 375°F/200°C.
2. Whisk the rice flour, tapioca starch, baking powder, salt, xanthan gum, garam masala, turmeric, cumin, sesame seeds, coconut milk and eggs together. Beat well until you have a smooth batter.
3. Pour the batter into a large freezer or food bag (this is done quite easily by placing the bag in a large glass and opening it up around and over the edges of the glass and pouring the batter in)
4. Careful snip a small corner off the bottom of the bag, holding on to the hole. Let go and allow the batter to pour

into the hot oil. Make sure you draw a "scribble" of the batter that crosses over itself to create a lattice type pattern, about 5-6" in diameter.

5. Cook for 2-3 minutes and then flip over and cook for a further 2-3 minutes until golden and cooked.

6. Drain on kitchen towel and repeat until all of the batter is used up.

7. Serve warm.

# Greek Salad Kebab (using the gluten-free snack loaf)

Serves 2

This great snack is healthy, gluten free and could make a great buffet dish. The salty feta is a lovely combination with the salad items and the gluten free bread really toasts well on the grill.

You could alter the vegetables depending on your preferences or what's available.

## **Ingredients**

- 4 plum tomatoes
- 8 olives
- 1 small courgette, cut into cubes
- 4 cubes of feta
- 4 large cubes of gluten-free bread (see recipe)
- 1 tbsp olive oil

**Instructions**

1. Using 4 metal skewers (you could use wooden ones but remember to soak them to prevent them from burning), thread the tomatoes, olives, courgette pieces, feta and bread on.

2. Drizzle over the olive oil.

3. Heat a griddle pan or grill and cook with a high heat until the vegetables are softened, and the feta and bread are a little charred.

# Toasted Welsh Rarebit (using the gluten-free snack loaf)

Serves 2

This classic super or dish uses the snack bread recipe, or you could use a gluten-free ready-made loaf. Traditionally made with flour, this has been made using arrowroot, but it still uses beer to give that lovely "yeasty" flavour. Make sure you use a gluten-free brew though!

## **Ingredients**

- 2 thick slices of gluten-free snack bread
- 1 tbsp arrowroot
- 1 tbsp butter
- ½ cup of beer
- ½ cup of strong cheddar cheese, grated
- 1 tsp English mustard
- 1 tbsp Worcestershire sauce

**Instructions**

1. Toast one side of the bread.

2. Meanwhile, heat the beer until simmering. Add the butter, mustard and Worcestershire sauce and stir until smooth.

3. Mix the arrowroot with a little water to make a paste and then add to the beer mix. Stir for a few minutes until thickened.

4. Stir in the grated cheese and keep mixing until it is melted, and the mixture is thick.

5. Spread on top of the untoasted side of bread.

6. Place under the grill and heat until golden and bubbling on top.

# Chicken Bombs and Chilli Dip

Serves: 4 as a snack

These little balls are great to store in the fridge and help yourself to when you're feeling a little peckish. They are made using chicken breast and make this a low fat, protein filled snack. Perfect as social gathering snack, there will be no need to discuss whether they are gluten-free (which of course they are!)

## **Ingredients**

- 1lb chicken breast mince (you could use turkey)
- 1 tsp olive oil
- 1 onion, chopped finely
- 1 garlic clove, crushed
- ¼ cup of ground almonds
- 1 tbsp dried oregano
- 1 tbsp nutritional yeast
- 1 egg, beaten

- 1 tsp salt

- 1-2 tbsp olive oil for cooking

- Sweet chilli sauce to serve

**Instructions**

1. Heat the oil in a frying pan and add the onion and garlic. Stir over a medium heat until they are soft but not coloured. Allow to cool a little.

2. Place the chicken mince, ground almonds, dried oregano, nutritional yeast and salt in a bowl and mix well. Add the egg and stir to combine thoroughly.

3. Using damp hands, make 20-25 small balls of the meat mix and place in the fridge to firm up a little.

4. Heat the oil in the frying pan to cook the meatballs. Add batches of the balls to the pan and cook for 6-7 minutes, turning over and browning on all sides. Repeat until all of the balls are cooked. You could bake these in the oven for an even healthier option.

5. Serve with a sweet chilli sauce to dip in, providing cocktail sticks.

# No-Cook Cracker Toppings Bonanza!

All Serve: 1

You can use any gluten-free cracker for these assembly only savoury snacks. No baking needed and it's a quick-to-prepare bite to eat when you're hungry.

## *The Hot Green One*

### Ingredients

- 2 large gluten-free crackers
- ½ avocado, stone removed and peeled
- 1 tbsp chopped fresh cilantro
- ¼ mild red chilli, diced finely, seeds removed

### Instructions

1. Place the crackers on a plate.

2. Mash the avocado with the cilantro and chilli.

3. Spread on to the crackers.

## *The Cheesy One*

### **Ingredients**

- 2 large gluten-free crackers
- 2 tbsp cream cheese
- 1 tbsp freshly grated parmesan cheese
- 1 spring onion, chopped

### **Instructions**

1. Place the crackers on a plate.
2. Spread the cream cheese on to the crackers.
3. Sprinkle the parmesan and spring onion on top.

## *The Italian One*

### **Ingredients**

- 2 large gluten-free crackers
- 5-6 olives
- 1 garlic clove, crushed
- 1 tbsp flat leaf parsley
- 2 baby plum tomatoes

### **Instructions**

1. Place the crackers on a plate.
2. Using a knife, chop the other ingredients together until really fine.
3. Spread on to the crackers and serve.

## *The Moroccan One*

### **Ingredients**

- 2 gluten-free crackers
- 2 tbsp ready-made houmous
- 1 tbsp toasted sesame seeds
- ¼ tsp ground cumin
- 3 dried apricots, chopped

### **Instructions**

1. Place the crackers on a plate.
2. Mix the houmous, cumin and apricots together.
3. Spread on to the crackers.
4. Top with the sesame seeds and serve.

# Smokey Cauliflower Steak

Serves 1

Cauliflower is such a handy ingredient to have in your fridge when you are following a gluten-free diet. It works well as a chunky steak what absorbs lots of flavour and this recipe could be increased or adapted further to add to a vegetarian main meal (may be with some grated cheese on).

## **Ingredients**

- 4 thick slices of cauliflower
- 1 tbsp olive oil
- ½ tsp smoked paprika
- 2 tbsps cornmeal
- ¼ tsp sea salt

**Instructions**

1. Pre-heat the oven to 400°F/200°C/Gas Mark 6 and grease or line a baking tray

2. Rub the olive oil all over the cauliflower and massage the paprika, cornmeal and salt in.

3. Place on the baking tray and bake for 15 minutes until softened and charred a little on top.

# Garlic Twists

Makes: 6-8 depending on the size you make!

These gluten-free sticks have lots of flavour and are great for snack, especially straight from the oven. Coconut flour is super absorbent, so add it 1 tablespoon at a time to see how much you will need.

## **Ingredients**

- 1 1/3 cups almond flour
- ½ tsp salt
- 3 tbsp coconut flour
- 2 tbsp coconut oil, melted
- 1 tsp garlic powder
- 1 tsp onion powder
- 3 eggs, beaten
- 1 tsp dried oregano
- 1 tsp dried thyme

- ½ tsp baking powder

- Melted butter for brushing

- 1 tbsp sesame seeds

**<u>Instructions</u>**

1. Pre-heat the oven to 400°F/200°C/Gas Mark 6 and grease a baking tray.

2. Place the oil and eggs in a bowl and mix well.

3. Add the almond flour, garlic powder, onion powder, salt, dried oregano, dried thyme and baking powder and stir well. Beat quite hard to make sure everything is as well combined.

4. Add the coconut flour, 1 tbsp at a time. Between each spoon, leave the dough for 5 minutes to see how much more you will need. You want to create a pliable dough that can be rolled out.

5. Cut the dough in to 6-8 equal pieces. Cut each of those pieces in to 3. Roll those three pieces into similar length sausages. Dab a little butter at the top to seal them and then plait the three sausages and seal again at the bottom. Do the same with all of the dough.

6. Place on the baking tray and brush with the melted butter.

7. Sprinkle over the sesame seeds and bake in the oven for 10-15 minutes until risen and golden.

8. Cool a little and devour!

# Smorgasbord

Serves 2

This is a great little "board" for when you are entertaining, and the guests are waiting for dinner. It also makes a rather luxurious TV snack to tuck in to when you're needing to fill in the gap between lunch and dinner, or even use it as a supper dish!

## **Ingredients**

- 2 slices of salami or other deli ham
- 8-10 olives, green or black or a mix
- 4-6 gluten-free breadsticks
- 6-8 cooked mini sausages
- 1 tsp wholegrain mustard (gluten free)
- 2 tsp honey
- Preheat the oven to 400°F/200°C/Gas Mark 6.

## Instructions

1. Mix the mustard, honey and sausages together and place in the oven, loosely wrapped in aluminium foil.

2. Find a wooden chopping board (or a plate) and place a little dish on it for the olives, a glass or cup for the breadsticks and keep a space for the ham.

3. Remove the sausages from the oven after about 10 minutes, you are just heating them through and glazing them, not cooking them. Put into a little bowl and place on the board with the other ingredients, ready to tuck in.

4. Note: This snack recipe could easily be doubled to feed more and use your imagination, fill the board with some lovely ingredients, just make sure they are all gluten-free.

# Bacon and Broccoli Fritter

Makes: 16

These little fritters are quick to prepare and full of vitamin C, vitamin K and folate. Make a batch up and keep in the fridge for when you find you have a hungry moment. They are delicious hot or cold and you could add some tomato and chilli salsa or garlic mayonnaise to top them if you like.

## Ingredients

- 2 medium heads of broccoli
- 1 onion, finely chopped
- 4 rashes of bacon, chopped
- 5 eggs, beaten
- ½ cup of almond flour
- 2 tbsp olive oil

## Instructions

1. Heat one tablespoon of the oil in a frying pan and cook the onion and bacon. Add to a bowl.

2. Roughly chop the broccoli and place in a food processor. Pulse until the broccoli is quite finely chopped and resembles rice. Add this to the bacon and onion.

3. Mix the beaten eggs and almond flour to the broccoli and make sure it is thoroughly combined.

4. Heat the other 1 tablespoon of oil in a frying pan and spoon the broccoli batter mix into mounds in the pan, but not over-crowding. Cook for 2-3 minutes on one side and then flip over to cook for another 2-3 minutes.

5. Repeat until all of the fritter mix has been used.

6. Serve warm or cold.

## *Energy Snacks*

When we need a snack, our body is crying out for energy or fuel so sometimes we need to fill it with good ingredients, especially if you have been training or using a lot of physical energy.

These snacks are all made with a protein of some sort and some have more than one source. You can always add extra protein powder for a bigger boost. Always ensure the powders you use are gluten-free and try and steer clear of any with added flavours and sweeteners.

Most of these energy snacks can be kept in an airtight container for 5-7 days which means you can be making these up once a week and you will always have a healthy snack available that your body will thank you for.

Take a note of the freezer fuel options, these can be kept frozen and eaten from frozen for 2 months after making and they are made with ingredients that are functional yet taste great.

# 3 Flavours of Energy

Each recipe makes 10

## *Chocolate Chip Energy Balls*

### **Ingredients**

- 1 ¼ cup of rolled oats (certified gluten free)
- 2 tbsp chia seeds
- ½ cup of peanut butter
- 1/3 cup of maple syrup
- 1 tsp vanilla extract
- ½ cup of dark chocolate chips

## *Cranberry and Honey Energy Balls*

- 1 ¼ cup of rolled oats (certified gluten free)
- 2 tbsp hemp seeds
- ½ cup of peanut butter

- 1/3 cup of honey
- ½ cup of dried cranberries

## *Bakewell Tart Energy Balls*

- 1 ¼ cup of rolled oats (certified gluten free)
- 2 tbsp flaxseed
- ½ cup of almond butter
- 1/3 cup of maple syrup
- 1 tsp almond extract/flavour
- ½ cup of freeze dried raspberries

## **Instructions**

1. Place all of the ingredients of the flavour you want to make into a mini food processor or blender and process until well combined but still a little chunky.
2. With damp hands, make approximately 10 balls of the mix and place in a plastic container.
3. Place in the fridge for 2 hours before consuming.

# Coconut Bounce Balls

Makes 15

Coconut is a great ingredient to use for energy. They are packed with vitamins and dietary fibre and they have a number of health benefits. Although high in fat, these particular fats are able to provide the body and brain with quick energy. They can raise the good HDL cholesterol in your blood that is linked to reducing heart disease and reduce the risk of stroke.

You can consume coconut water, milk, cream, flesh (desiccated or flaked), oil and butter and all are really useful in gluten-free baking.

## **Ingredients**

- 1 cup of desiccated coconut, unsweetened
- 1 cup of cashews
- ¼ cup of sunflower seeds
- ¼ cup of whole almonds

- 2 tbsp cacao nibs

- Pinch of salt

- ½ cup coconut butter, melted

- ½ cup of coconut oil, melted

- 3 tbsp maple syrup or yacon syrup

## **Instructions**

1. Place all of the ingredients into a mini food processor or blender and process until well combined but still a little chunky.

2. With damp hands, make approximately 15 balls of the mix and place in a plastic container.

3. Place in the fridge for 2 hours before consuming.

# Middle Eastern Boost

Makes: 10

Tahini is used in this recipe as one of the binders. It is made from sesame seeds and a great source of protein, magnesium, manganese and copper.

## **Ingredients**

- 2 cups walnuts
- 1 cup desiccated unsweetened coconut
- 1 cups soft Medjool dates, pitted
- ½ cup of tahini
- 2 tablespoons coconut oil
- 1/2 teaspoon sea salt
- 1 teaspoon vanilla extract
- A splash of water if needed

## **Instructions**

1. Place all of the ingredients into a mini food processor or blender and process until well combined but still a little chunky.

2. With damp hands, make approximately 10 balls of the mix and place in a plastic container.

3. Place in the fridge for 2 hours before consuming.

# Freezer Fuel

Each recipe makes: 10

These two freezer fuels are a great idea to keep in the freezer for those moments when you need a "pick me up". They are far better than reaching for a bag of crisps or chocolate bar and they take minutes to prepare.

Store in the freezer in an air tight container for up to 2 months.

## **Ingredients**

- Fudgy Chocolate
- ½ cup pecans
- 15 Medjool dates, roughly chopped
- 1/3 cup of desiccated coconut
- 1 tbsp coconut oil
- 2 tbsp cocoa powder

- White Chocolate

- ½ cup of cashews

- 4 oz white chocolate, softened

- 10 Medjool dates, roughly chopped

- 1/3 cup of desiccated coconut

- 1 tbsp coconut oil

- 1 tbsp coconut butter, softened

### **Instructions**

1. Place all of the ingredients of the flavour you want to make into a mini food processor or blender and process until well combined but still a little chunky.
2. With damp hands, make approximately 10 balls of the mix and place in a plastic container.
3. Place in the freezer for at least 2 hours before consuming.

## Sticky Date Energy Bars

Makes: 8

These bars are so easy to make and are gloriously sweet. No added sugars, they are sweetened with just the dried fruits and will give you a burst of energy.

Almonds are a great source of vitamins, minerals and protein and will provide you with fibre, magnesium and the hormone balancing, vitamin E.

## **Ingredients**

- 1 cup of whole almonds
- 1 cup of dried cranberries or raisins
- 1 cup of pitted dates
- 2 tbsp desiccated coconut
- 1 tbsp chia seeds

## Instructions

1. Line a small baking tray with cling film.
2. Place all of the ingredients into a mini-processor or blender and pulse until the mix is quite fine and broken down.
3. Press down into the baking tray to make a ½" thick rectangle.
4. Place in the fridge for at least 2 hours.
5. Remove from the fridge and peel away from the cling film.
6. Cut the rectangle into 8 bars.
7. These are best stored in the fridge as they can be a little sticky.

# Tropical Energy Bars

Makes: 10

These flavours will evoke thoughts of faraway shores of white sand and crystal-clear waters. Coconut, apricot, peaches and vanilla are all added to this recipe, along with a pinch of all spice.

By soaking the cashew nuts beforehand, you will create a lovely soft textured bar that adds a little creaminess to some gluten-free energy.

## **Ingredients**

- ½ cup of dried apricots
- ½ cup of dried peaches
- ½ cup cashews (soaked overnight in water and drained)
- ½ cup desiccated coconut
- ½ cup rolled oats
- 1 tsp vanilla extract

- 2 tbsp agave syrup or yacon syrup

- 2 tbsp chia seeds

- Pinch of allspice powder

- ½ tsp dried ginger

## **Instructions**

1. Place all of the ingredients into a food processor or high-speed blender and pulse until all the ingredients are finely chopped and combined.

2. Line a small baking tray with cling film and press the mix into the tin.

3. Place in the fridge for at least 2 hours.

4. Remove and peel away from the cling film. Cut in to 10 bars and store in the fridge for 5-7 days.

# Bike Bites

Makes: 24 bite sized chunks

These are great for cycling enthusiasts and full of a mix of energy enhancing seeds.  If you are riding a long session it is vital that you take in adequate hydration and nutrition or you will be at risk of injury.  These bike bars are perfect to store in a bike pack and can easily be cut into chunks that you can grab and graze on during the ride.  They are firm enough to stick together and can be made up to 7 days ahead.

## **Ingredients**

- 1 cup of pumpkin seeds
- ½ cup of sunflower seeds
- ½ cup of sesame seeds
- 4 tbsp hemp seeds, shelled
- 1 cup of dried dates
- 6 tbsp coconut oil, melted
- 3 tbsp cocoa powder

- 3 tbsp chia seeds
- 5 tbsp rolled oats

## **Instructions**

1. Place all of the ingredients into a food processor or high-speed blender. Process until the mix is quite finely chopped.
2. Line a small baking tray with cling film and press the mix down well.
3. Place in the fridge for at least 2 hours. Remove and peel away from the cling film.
4. Cut in to bite sized chunks and store in the fridge until you're ready to ride.

## Peanut Butter Energy Cups

Makes: 9

These are quite similar to the peanut butter cups you can buy, but without all the processed sugars and they are guaranteed to be gluten-free and full of energy. Use any gluten-free protein powder for this and make sure the oats are certified gluten-free.

### **Ingredients**

- 1 cup of rolled oats
- ½ cup of oat flour
- 3 scoops of protein powder of your choice
- ½ cup of popped rice cereal
- ¼ cup of maple syrup
- ½ cup of peanut butter
- 1 tsp vanilla extract
- 1 tbsp cocoa powder
- 3 tbsp dark chocolate chips

## Instructions

1. Place all of the ingredients, except the chocolate chips, into a food processor or high-speed blender and process until quite smooth. Mix the chocolate in as best you can, this will be quite stiff, so you could briefly "pulse" your machine, but be careful not to break the chocolate up too much as you still want it nice and chunky

2. Line a small baking tray with cling film. Press the mixture into the tin and place in the fridge for 2 hours.

3. Cut into 9 bars and keep in the fridge in an airtight container for 5-7 days.

# Apple Pie Energy Bars

Makes 16

There is always a smile when apple pie flavours are about. Cinnamon and soft sweet apples with all the buttery comfort of the pastry is replicated in this energy bar. Ground almonds replace the pastry and the apple sauce is the main sweetener. Walnuts have been added to give a good boost of energy from the protein and good fats they contain.

## **Ingredients**

- 2 cps of rolled oats
- 1 cup of ground almonds
- 1 cup of walnuts, chopped
- ¼ cup of maple syrup
- 1 tsp ground cinnamon
- ½ cup of unsweetened apple sauce
- 1 tsp vanilla extract
- 1 tbsp almond butter

## Instructions

1. Place all of the ingredients into a food processor or high-speed blender and process until the mix is quite fine and combined,

2. Line a small baking tray with cling film and press the mixture into it.

3. Place in the fridge for 2 hours to cool.

4. Remove from the fridge and peel away the cling film. Cut in to 16 slices and store in an airtight container.

# Ginger Rush Bars

Makes 12

The stem ginger in syrup is used for this recipe (there are others in this book so don't waste it!) and adds a great sweet ginger flavour without too much of the heat. Add the chopped nuts and ginger in after processing as these will give the bars a lovely crunch and texture.

## **Ingredients**

- 1 cup of rolled oats
- ½ cup of cornflakes
- ¼ cup of desiccated coconut
- 1/3 cup of almond butter
- ¼ cup maple syrup
- 1 tbsp hemp seeds
- ½ cup of Medjool dates
- 1 ball of stem ginger, chopped

- 4 tbsp roughly chopped almonds

## **Instructions**

1. Place the rolled oats, cornflakes, desiccated coconut, almond butter, maple syrup, hemp dates, and dates in a food processor or a high-speed blender and process until finely chopped. Stir through the ginger and almonds.

2. Line a small baking tray with cling film and press the mixture in. Place in the fridge for 2 hours until firm.

3. Remove from the fridge and peel away the cling film.

4. Cut the bar in to 12 slices.

# Fudge Brownie Energy Bar

Makes 12

Rather like a fudge brownie but without any gluten and a whole load of processed sugars, this energy bar will appeal to the chocoholics. The base uses black beans, and this provides a great boost of energy. These are also nut-free, so if you do suffer with allergies or eat with others with allergies, this would be a great alternative to the nut heavy energy bars out there.

## **Ingredients**

- 1 ½ cup of tinned black beans, drained and rinsed well
- 4 tbsp cocoa powder
- 7 tbsp protein powder of choice
- 1/3 cup of maple syrup
- 3 ½ tbsp coconut oil, melted
- 1 tbsp vanilla extract
- ½ tsp baking powder (gluten-free)
- 1/3 cups of dark chocolate chips (at least 70% cocoa)

## **Instructions**

1. Pre-heat the oven to 375°F/190°C/Gas Mark 5 and grease or line a small baking tray.

2. Place all of the ingredients, except the chocolate chips, into a food processor or high-speed blender and process until really smooth.

3. Stir in the chocolate chips and press into the prepared baking tray.

4. Place in the oven and bake for 20 minutes maximum. Be careful not to overcook as the stodgier and softer this bake is, the better! They will look undercooked when you remove them but place them in the fridge to firm up and you will easily be able to cut the bakes into 12 bars.

## Nut Free Energy Balls

Makes: 15

Many of the recipes for energy bars contain nuts, which is a real problem if you are avoiding gluten and nuts. This recipe is perfect for a hit of energy and uses sunflower butter to add a great nut-free "nutty" taste!

### **Ingredients**

- 1 cup of dates
- 1/3 cup of coconut oil, melted
- 2 scoops of protein powder
- 2/3 cup of oat flour
- 2 tbsp flaxseeds
- 1/3 cup of sunflower seeds
- 1/3 cup of pumpkin seeds
- ¼ cup of desiccated coconut
- 3 tbsp sunflower seeds butter

- 1 tsp vanilla extract

## **Instructions**

1. Place all of the ingredients into a food processor or high-speed blender and process until fine.

2. Using damp hands, squeeze the mix in to 15 balls and store in the fridge. Add a little more sunflower seed butter or maple syrup if the mix is a little dry as it will depend on how soft your dates are. The pitted Medjool dates are the biggest and juiciest of dates to use.

Before you go, I'd like to remind you that there is a free, complimentary eBook waiting for you. Download it today to treat yourself to healthy, <u>gluten-free desserts and snacks</u> so that you never feel deprived again!

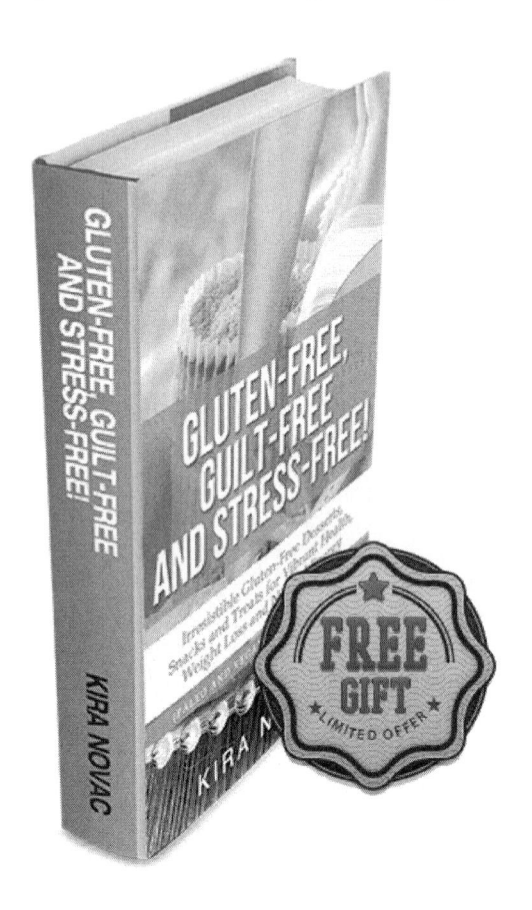

**Download link**

http://bit.ly/gluten-free-desserts-book

# Conclusion

There are many reasons to follow a gluten-free diet nowadays and it is now much easier to achieve than even just a few years ago. With a wealth of gluten-free products available and even shop shelves dedicated to them, you can readily buy snacks and cooked items, so you don't have to try to bake or make them yourselves.

With gluten-free flours and breads having much bad press over the years, baking at home was never really considered by many as success was limited. Many gluten-free bakers can probably own up to a few disasters of inedible results. However, along with all of these gluten-free ready-made items, we are now finding a growing number of emerging flours, seeds and grains becoming available to us and this has ended up with many more of us experimenting with cooking at home. Tasty alternatives are being made and this diet is now much easier to manage and can be really good for us. It is useful to remember though, gluten-free does not necessarily mean healthy! A gluten-free donut that has been deep fried and coated in a thick layer of sugar is still not a staple for everyday!

Gluten-free bakes do seem to come with a premium, so it is really worth trying to find your favourite flour blends and recipes to both save money and help you avoid processed foods. If these recipes have inspired you to get cooking but you are the only gluten-free member in your household, you can freeze ready-portioned items for easy removal or get everyone else to eat them too!

By avoiding gluten, many of us find digestive issues and symptoms can be eased or resolved and this is great for your gut. We should all be eating many different sources of food, colours and textures to improve our gut health and to get the best, all round nutrition possible and by experimenting with different bases and grains you can really improve your overall health.

Gluten-free is not just for allergies, coeliac's and health problems, it's for those who love creating healthy, imaginative and tasty dishes and most of all, it's for everyone who loves food.

## To post an honest review

One more thing... If you have received any value from this book, can you please rank it and post a short review? It only takes a few seconds really and it would really make my day. It's you I am writing for and your opinion is always much appreciated. In order to do so;

1. Log into your account
2. Search for my book on Amazon or check your orders/ or go to my author page at:

<u>http://amazon.com/author/kira-novac</u>

3. Click on a book you have read, then click on "reviews" and "create your review".

Please let me know your favorite motivational tip you learned from this book.

I would love to hear from you!

If you happen to have any questions or doubts about this book, please e-mail me at:

kira.novac@kiraglutenfreerecipes.com

I am here to help!

# Recommended Reading

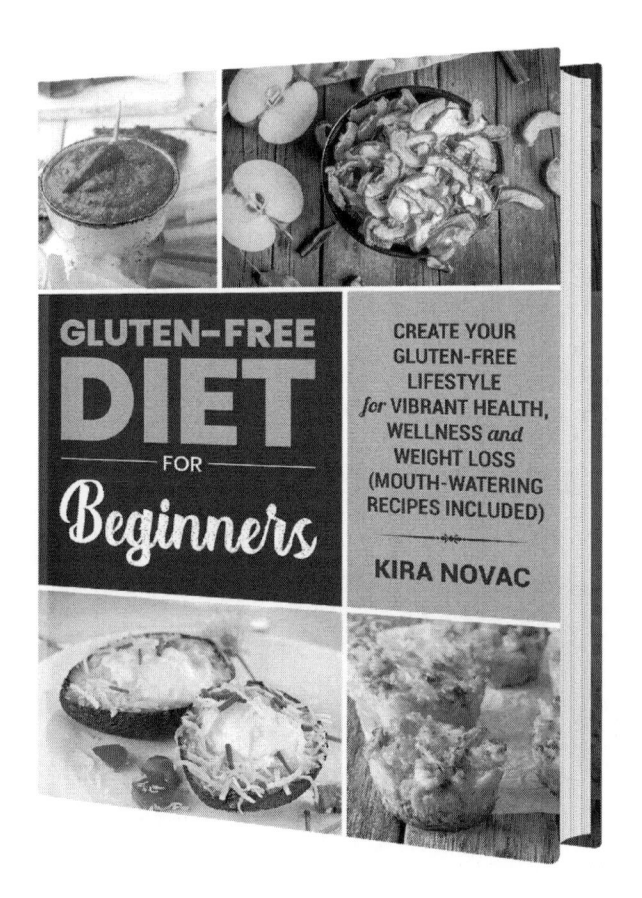

Buy it here:

http://bit.ly/gf-beginners

# Recommended Reading

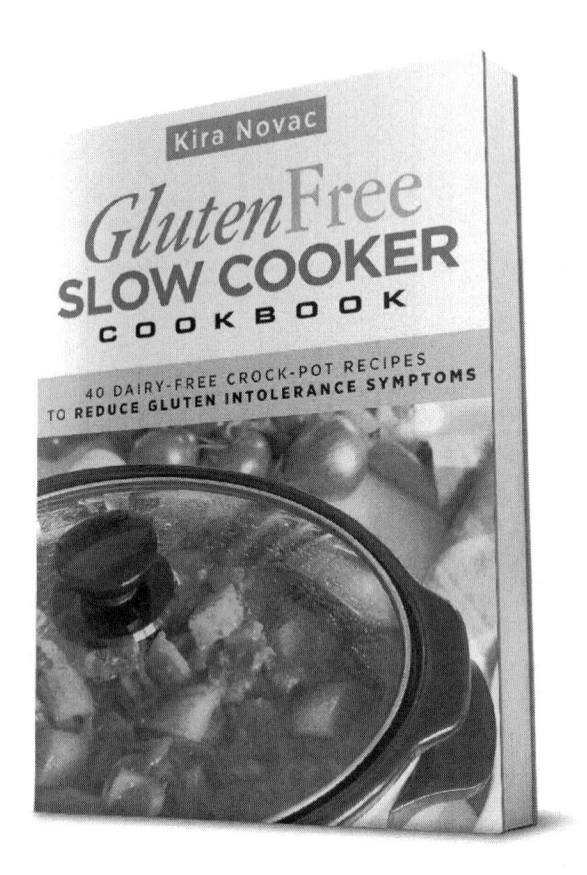

Buy it here:

http://bit.ly/gf-slow

# For More Gluten-Free Books (Kindle & Paperback) By Kira Novac, Please Visit:

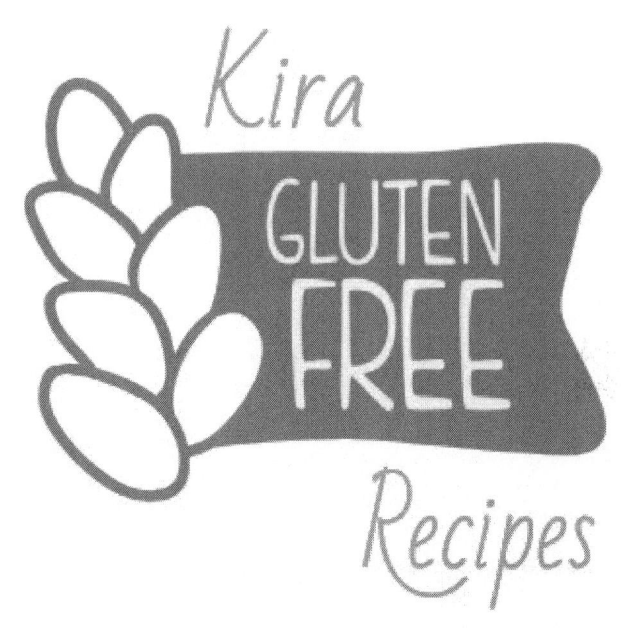

**www.kiraglutenfreerecipes.com/books**

Thank you for taking an interest in my work,

Kira Novac

Printed in Poland
by Amazon Fulfillment
Poland Sp. z o.o., Wrocław